THE BOOK OF HEARTS

Robert Delpire et Andrē Martin

WARNER BOOKS

A Warner Communications Company

Warner Books Edition
Copyright c 1977 by Warner Books, Inc. All rights reserved
ISBN 0-446-87495-7
Warner Books Inc., 75 Rockefeller Plaza, New York, N.Y. 10019
Printed in France
Not associated with Warner Press, Inc., of Anderson, Indiana
First Printing September 1977
A Warner Communications Company

Jan 1978

for the
tender heart ....

.... to Shelley

Happy Birthday   Love Clyde

Introduction

The dictionary definition of a heart is: 'Hollow organ keeping up circulation by contracting and dilating'. It weighs about 260 grammes.

Revealed by a surgeon, it gleams in its lustrous red sheath and pumps with a heavy sustained vigour. A dull, obstinate organ, doing its job, it bears little more physical resemblance to the hearts scrawled on walls or carved on trees by lovers than does the Chinese character for heart, XIN.

From one culture to another, the symbol used to denote a heart has been different; in ancient Egypt, an urn; among primitives, an 'oeil du coeur'.

These symbols are so ancient they owe their origins to a period before the invention of the written word; and yet they have survived its invention; ideograms, pictograms, glyphs, hieroglyphs.

They had little to do with the raw hearts warriors once plucked from their fallen victims' breasts or, over which in the most modern operating theatres surgeons now pause, knife in hand.

They were never intended to be portraits of a sinewy, heaving muscle, the size of a clenched fist. The symbols were symptoms of life, a kind of instantly accessible mental shorthand; a vestless motif, found on wells, in dungeons, in bakers' moulds, in pendants, a design used by tattooists; or represented garlanded with roses or bound with thorns, pierced by arrows, by daggers; nothing to do with the real heart; the heart that just went on beating, mindless as a metronome.

They were stand-ins for the real heart, a heartless watch that kept a time so accurate it could never be celebrated on any scale but its own; time only to flux; a watch that would one day stop.

The dictionary definition continues: 'seat of the emotions or affections; soul; mind'. If the images retain a spontaneity that words lack (though commemorated in language in phrases like 'light-hearted', 'broken-hearted', 'cold-hearted', 'sweetheart' and so on) it is perhaps because, in a universe without heart, each of its inhabitants has one, and, willingly or unwillingly, shares in a single heartbeat.

Claude Roy
Adapted by Peter Stark

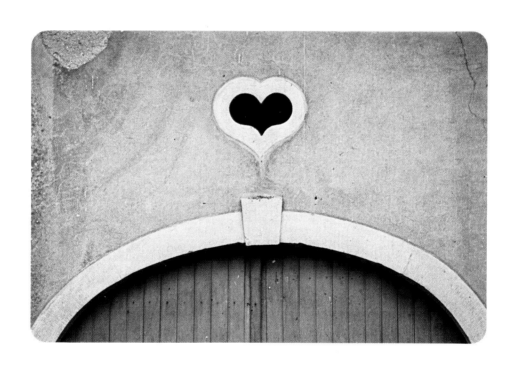

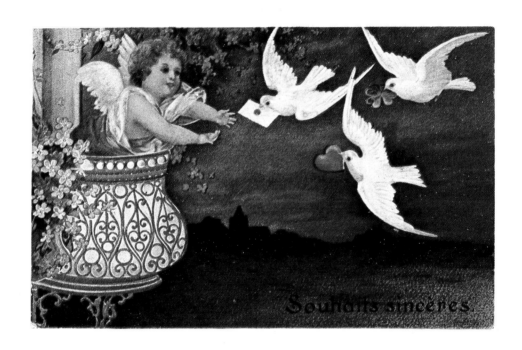

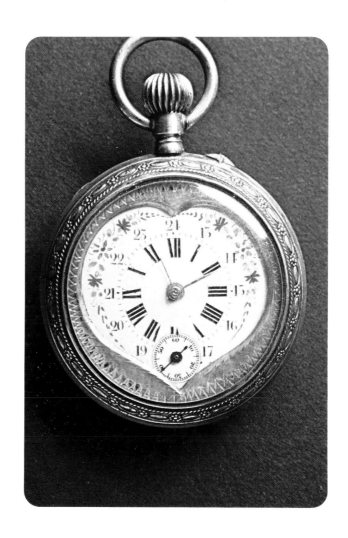

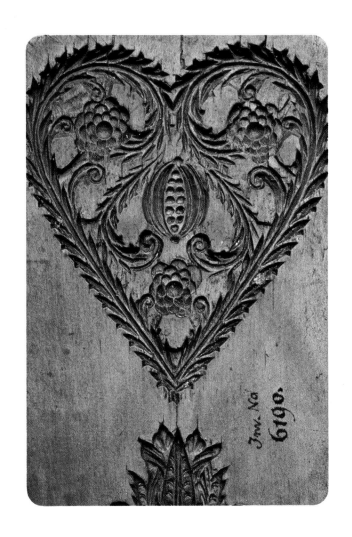

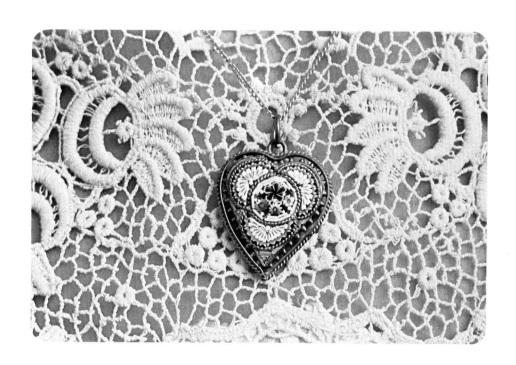

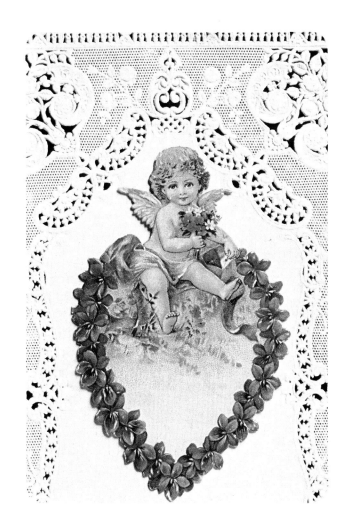

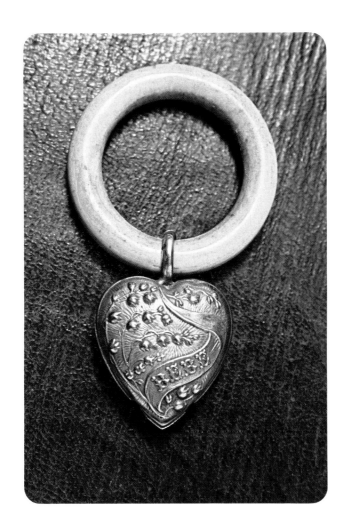

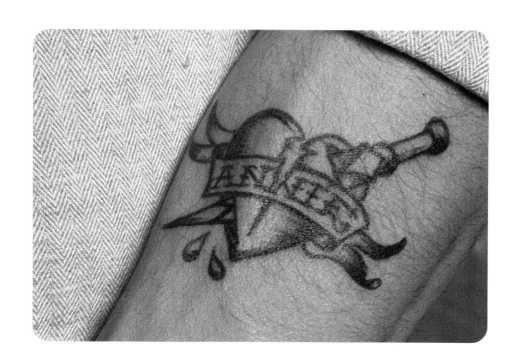

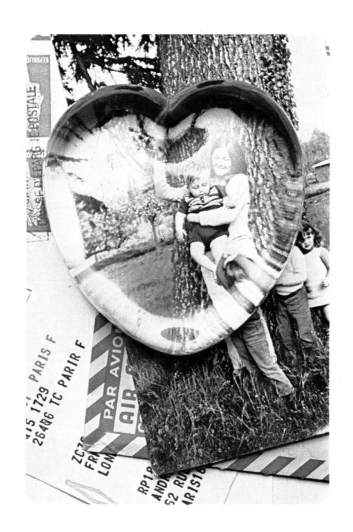

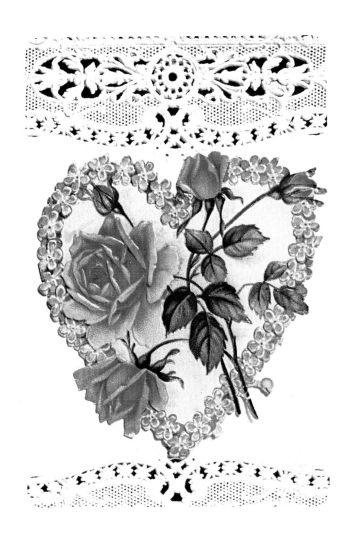

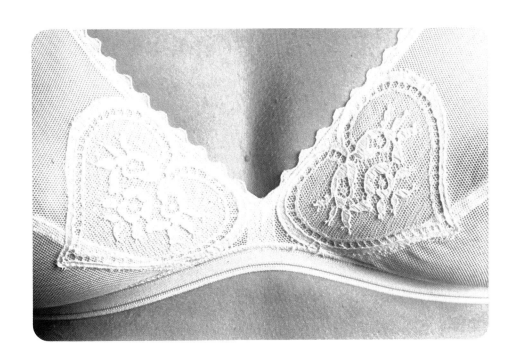

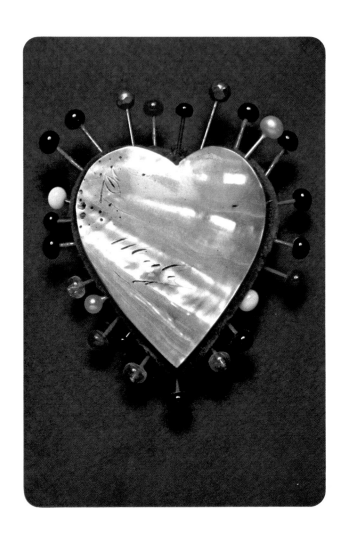

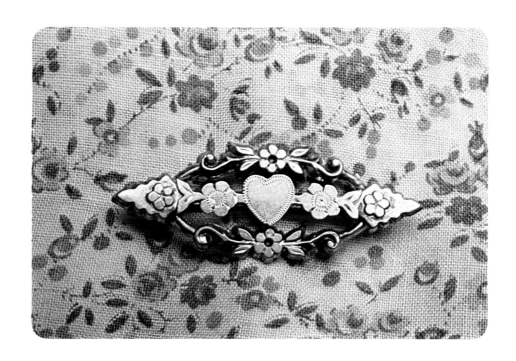

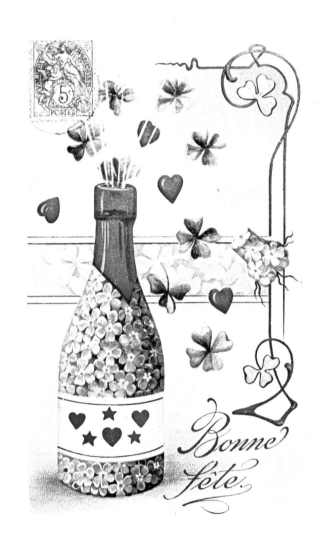

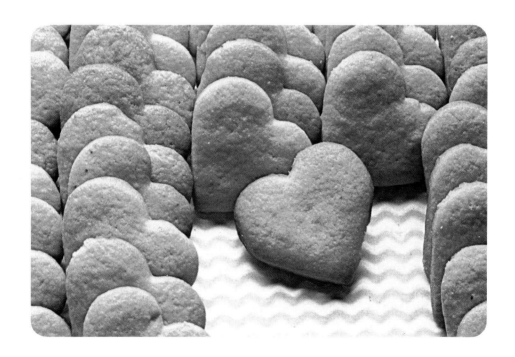

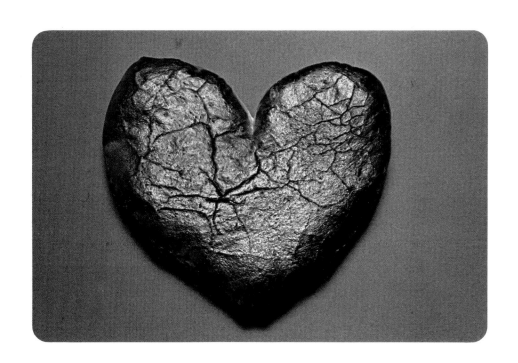

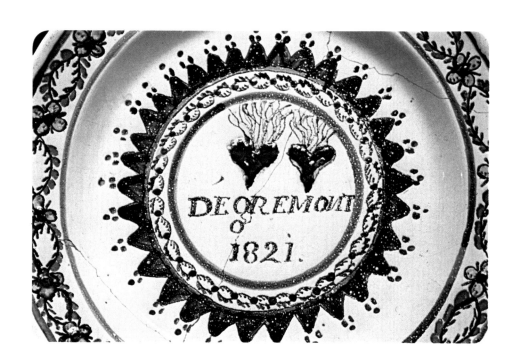

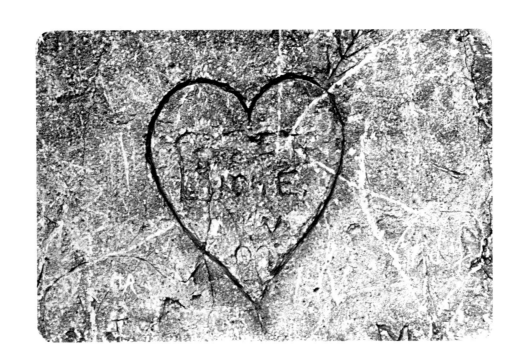

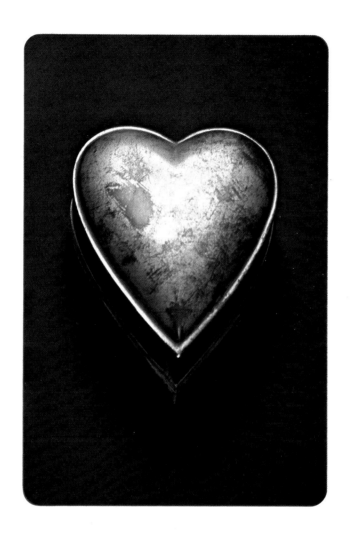

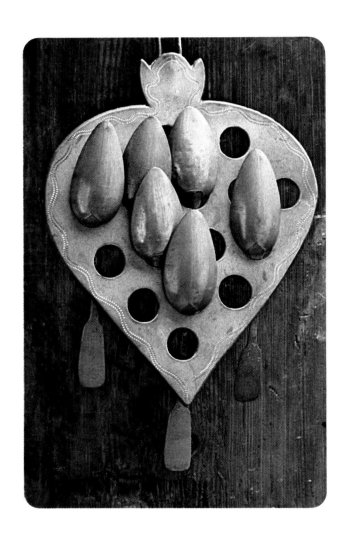

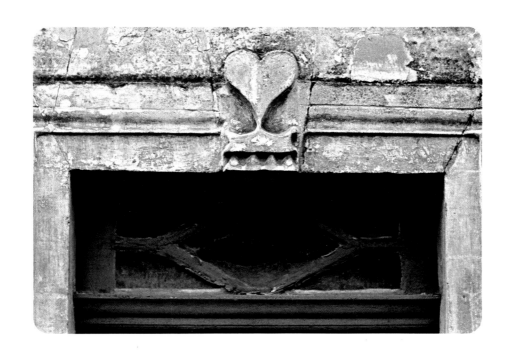

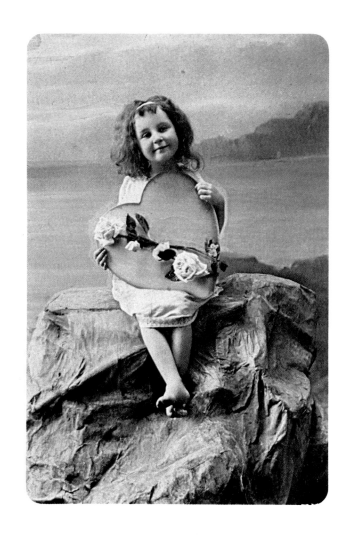

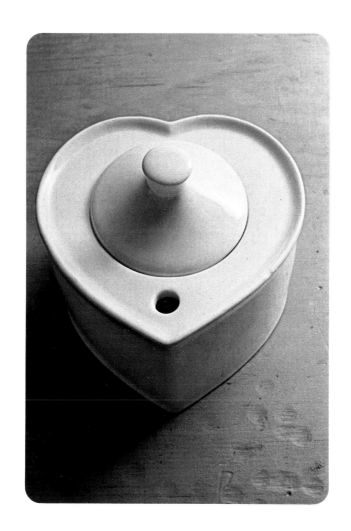

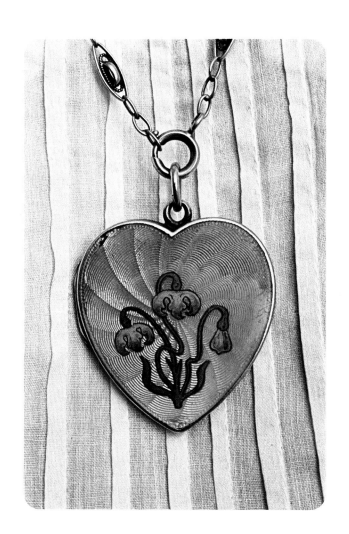

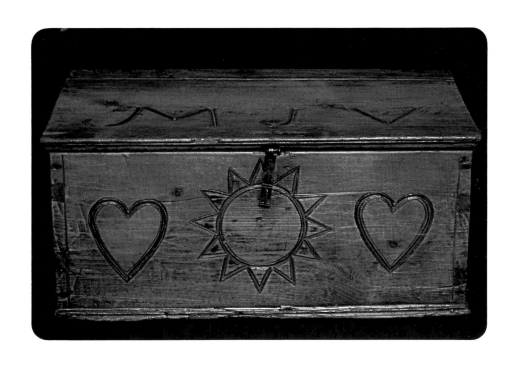

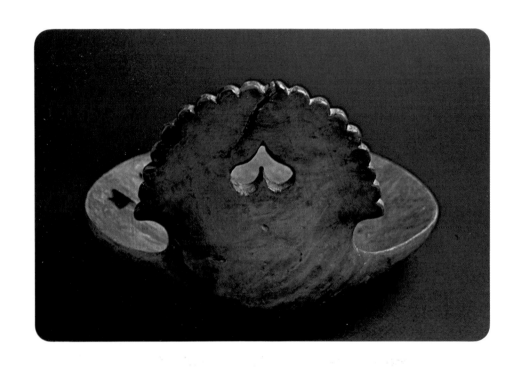

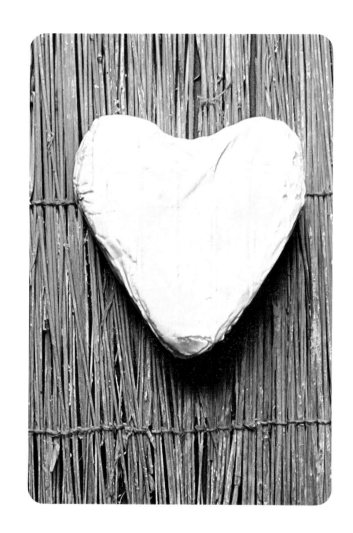

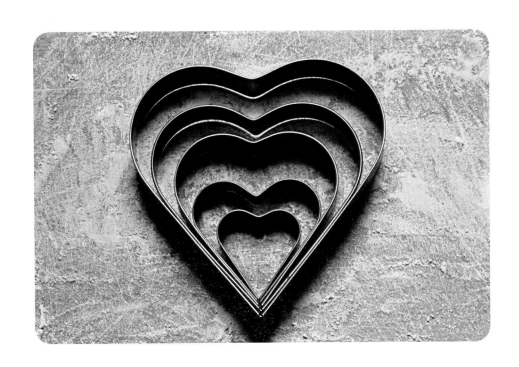

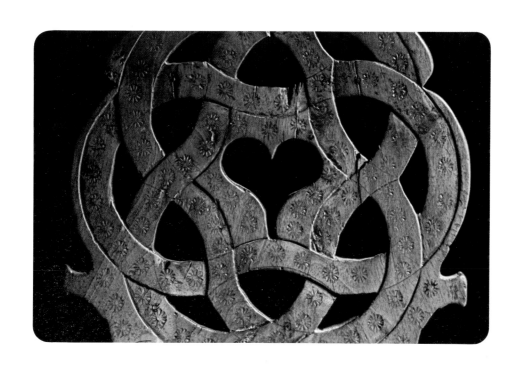

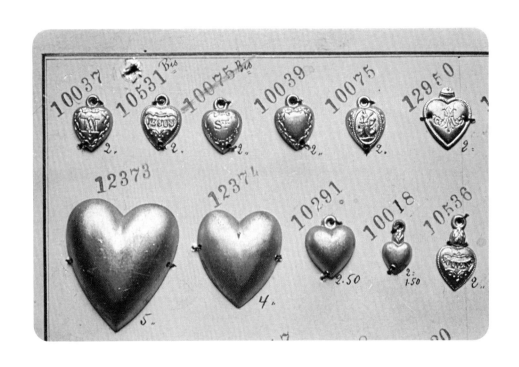

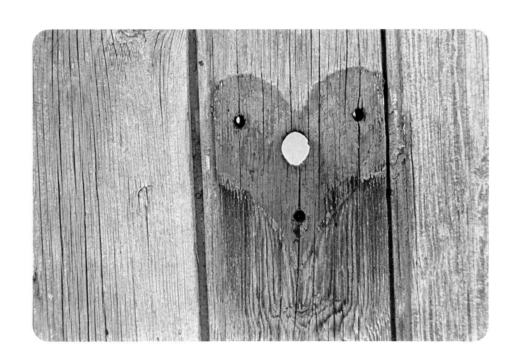

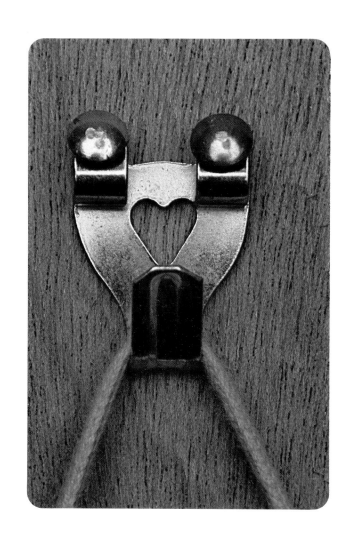

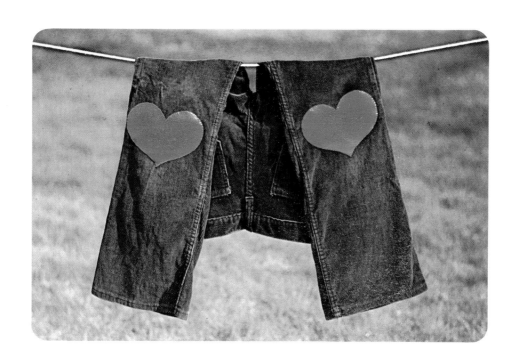

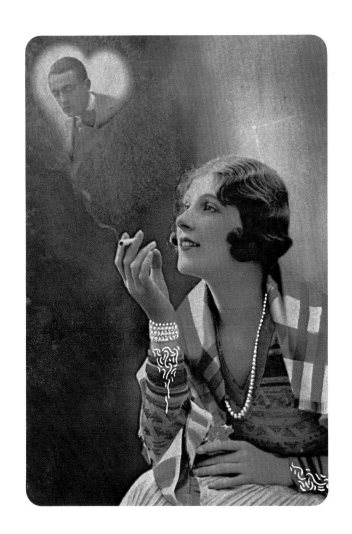

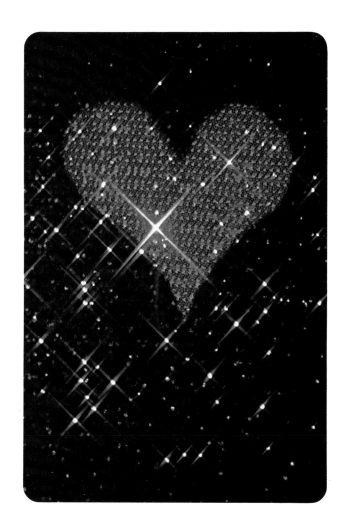

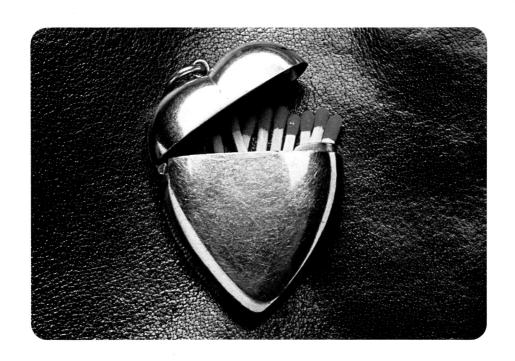

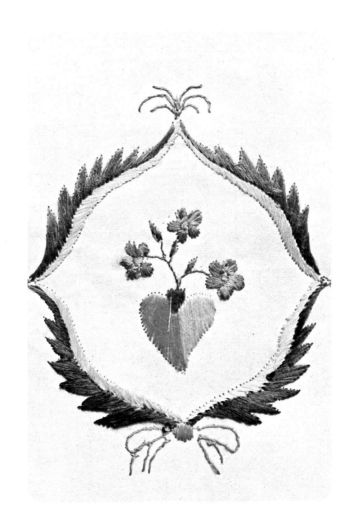

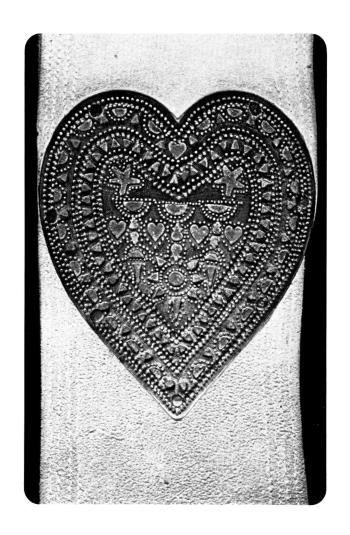

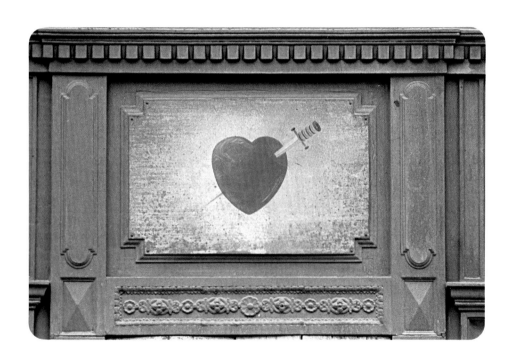

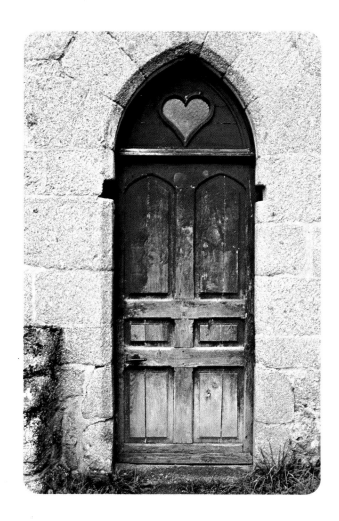

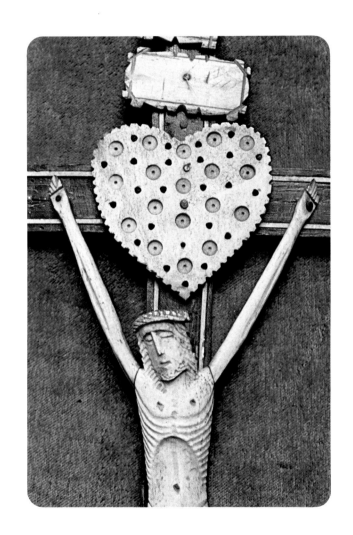

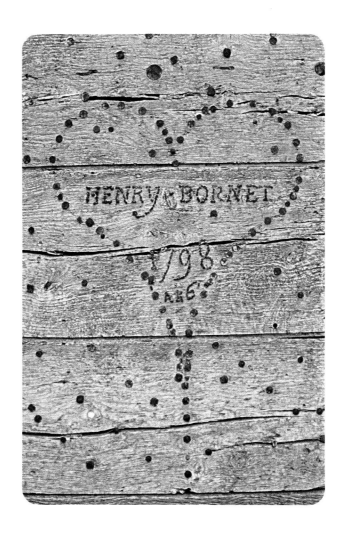

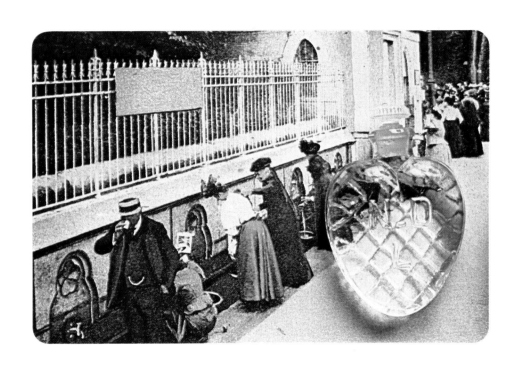

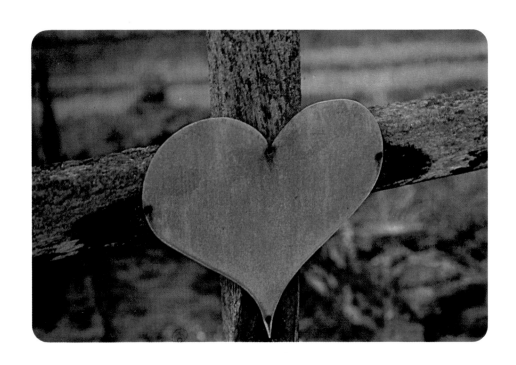

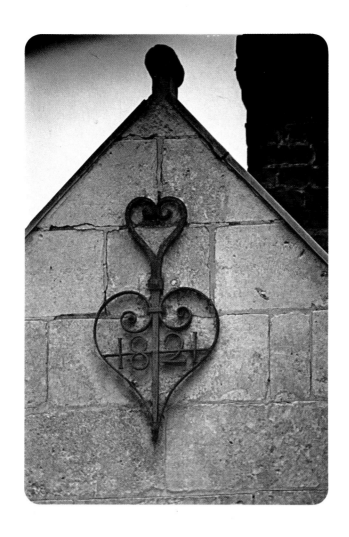

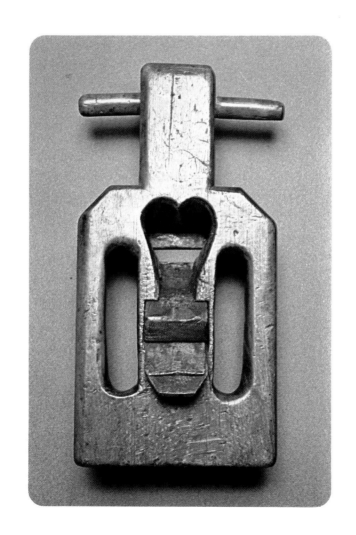

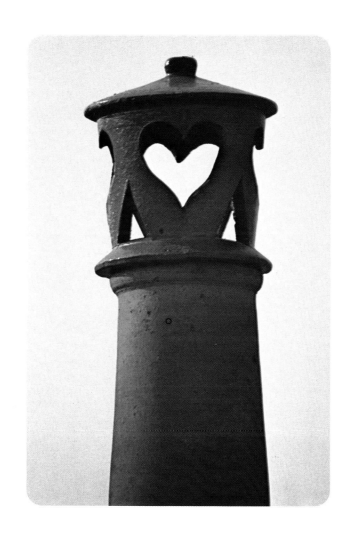

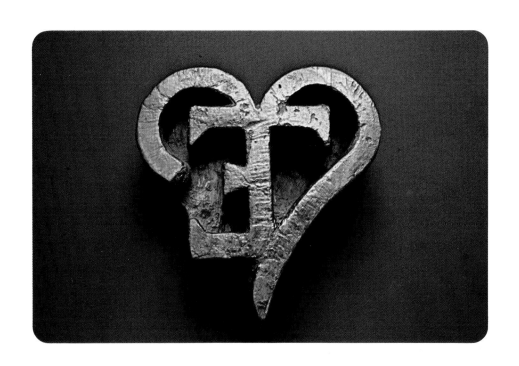

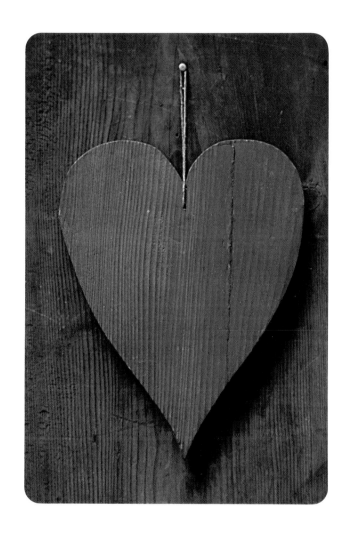

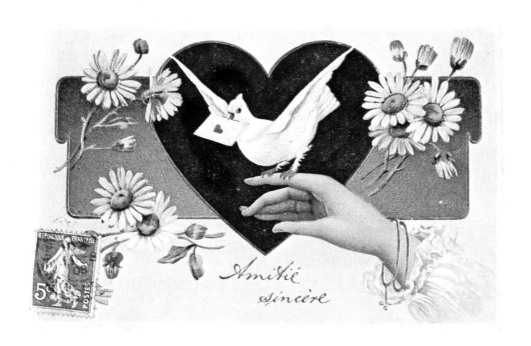

Amitié
sincère

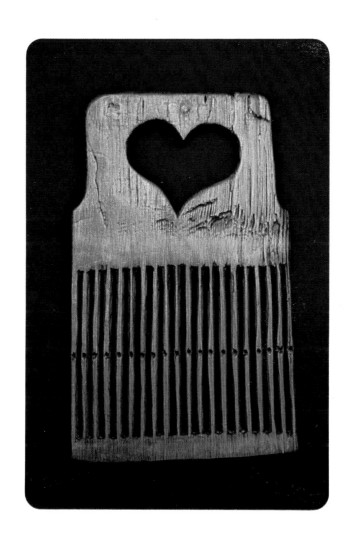

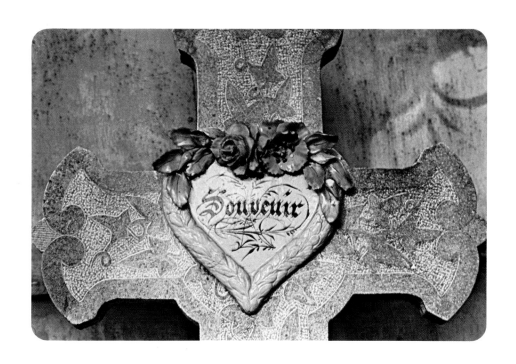

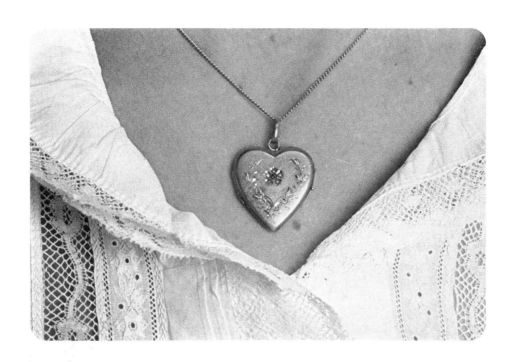

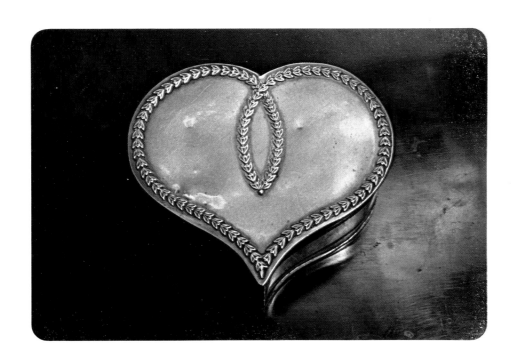

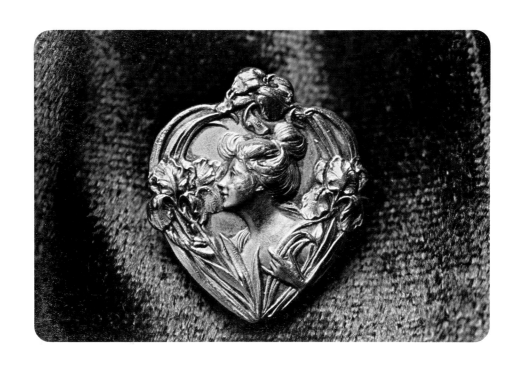

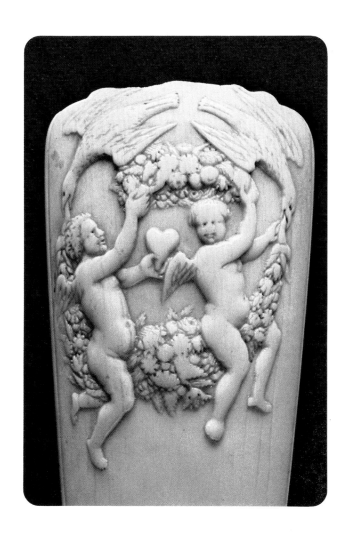

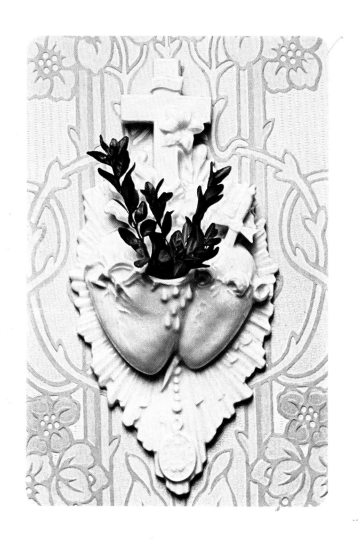

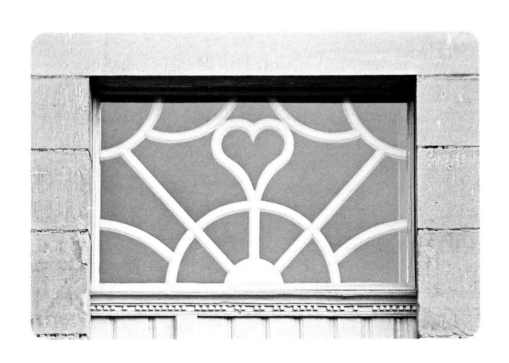

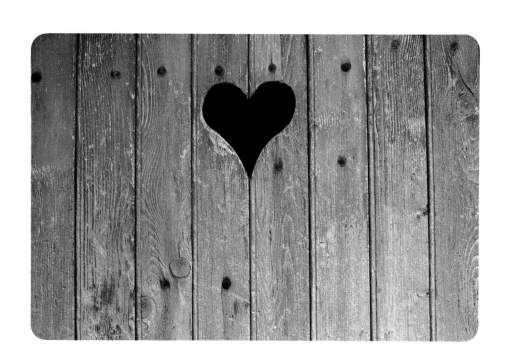

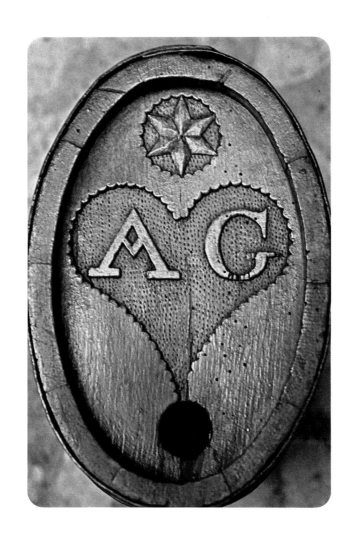

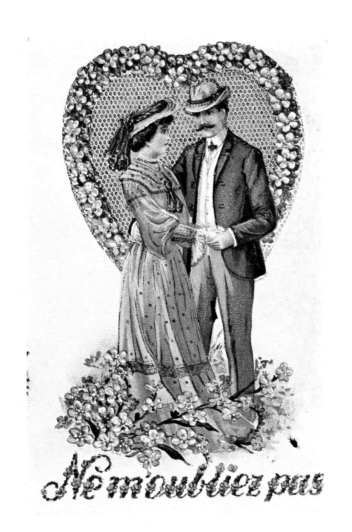

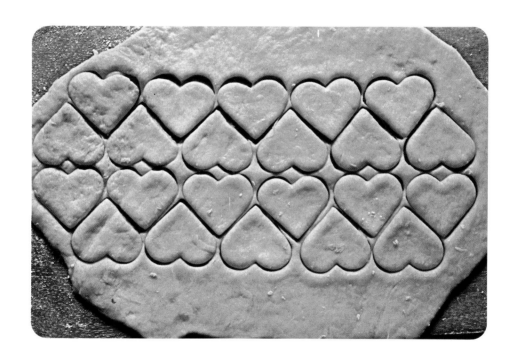

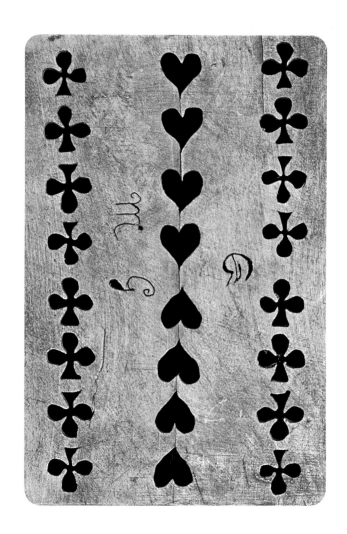

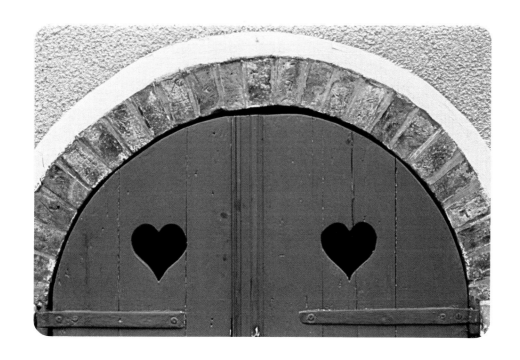

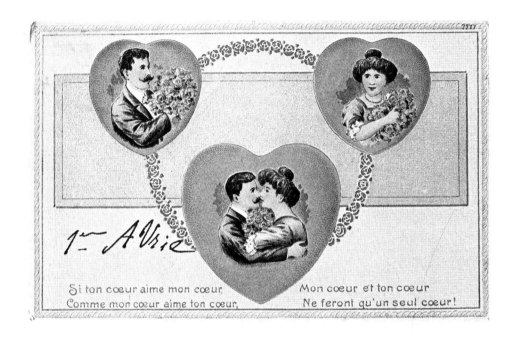

1ᵉʳ Avril

Si ton cœur aime mon cœur,   Mon cœur et ton cœur
Comme mon cœur aime ton cœur,   Ne feront qu'un seul cœur!

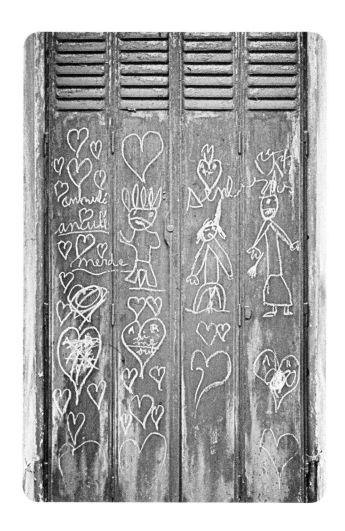

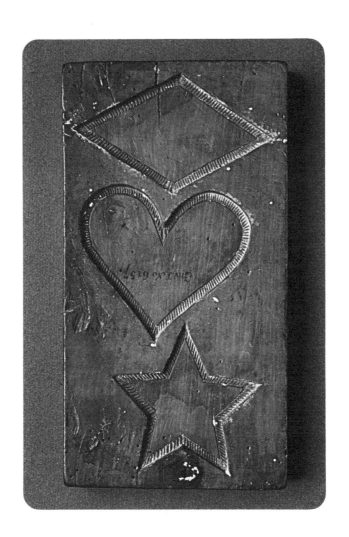

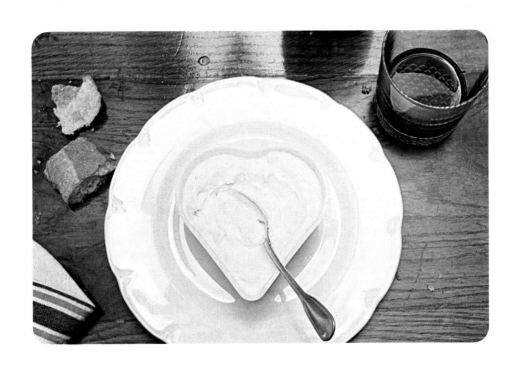

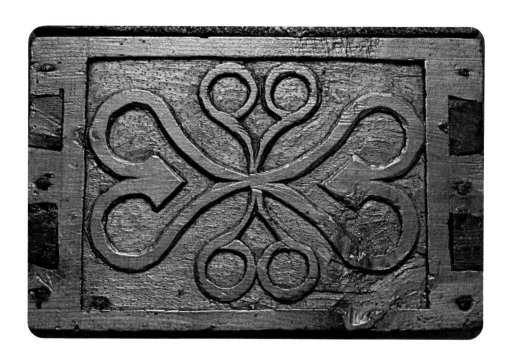

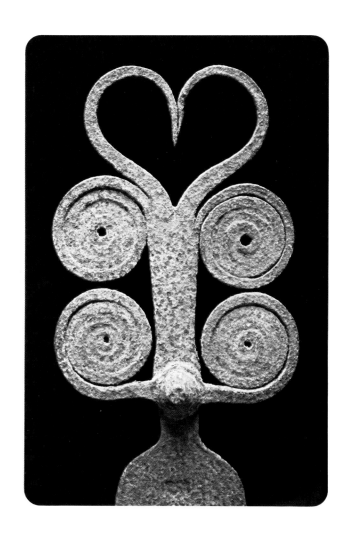

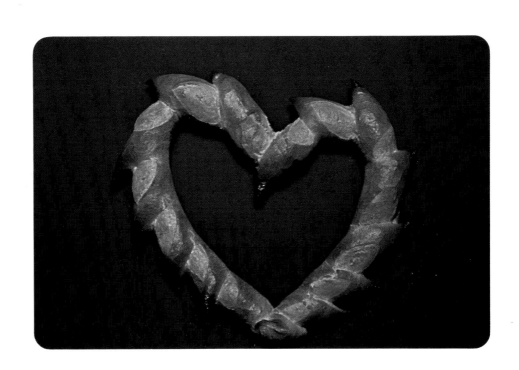

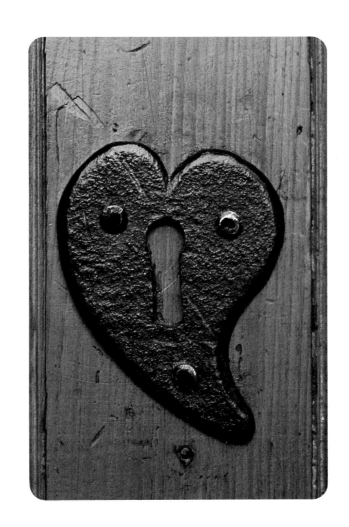

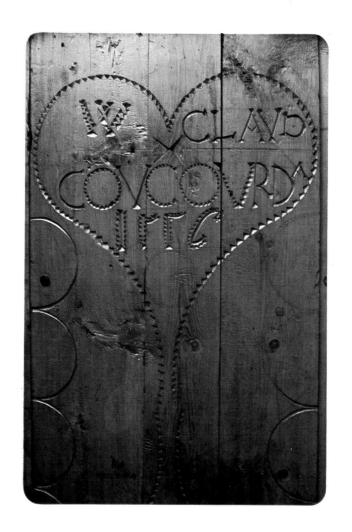

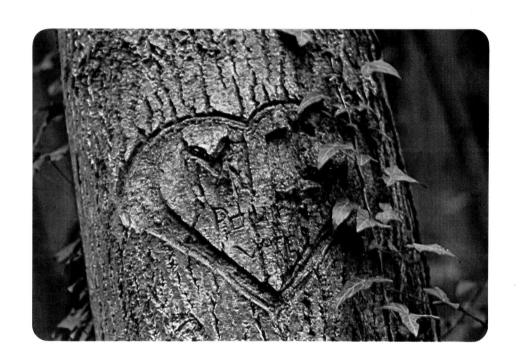

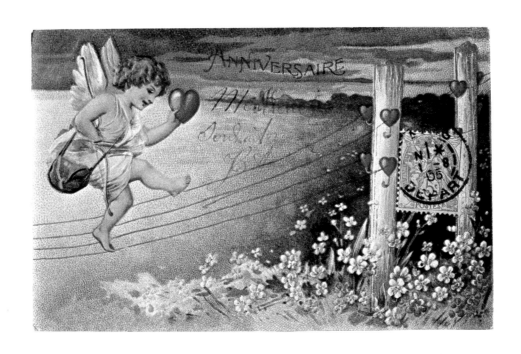